Female Nourishment and Hormones

A way to obtain hormonal stability, shed weight and feel alive.

By

Gold M. Crown

Table of contents

Introduction

The world of hormones.

Hormones are chemical messengers which are secreted immediately into the blood, which incorporates them into organs and tissues of the frame to exert their functions. There are many types of hormones that act on distinct elements of bodily functions and procedures. Some of those encompass:

Development and growth

Metabolism of meals items

Sexual function and reproductive boom and fitness

Cognitive function and temper

Maintenance of frame temperature and thirst

Where are they secreted from?

Hormones are secreted from the endocrine glands inside the frame. The glands are ductless, so hormones are secreted at once into the bloodstream rather than by way of ducts. Some of the principal endocrine glands inside the body consist of:

Pituitary gland

Pineal gland

Thymus

Thyroid

Adrenal glands

Pancreas

Testes

Ovaries

These organs secrete hormones in microscopic amounts and it takes the simplest very small amounts to result in essential adjustments within the body. Even a slight extra of hormone secretion can result in ailment states, as can the slightest deficiency in a hormone.

Hormones are also chemical messengers that help your cells communicate and trigger diverse actions. They're the bedrock of your frame's endocrine gadget, which regulates growth, reproduction, metabolism, temperature, or even your temper.

Hormones and the endocrine gadget maintain your frame in a balanced nation of homeostasis. Therefore, having a hormonal imbalance of too little or too much of a sure hormone can have dangerous facet outcomes.

Oxidative pressure, infertility, and endocrine disorders like thyroid disorder are just a few conditions that could result from hormonal imbalances.

Women undergo herbal changes to their hormone tiers at sure instances all through their lifecycle, substantially during puberty, being pregnant, and menopause.

Similarly, guys may additionally revel in symptoms of hormonal imbalances throughout puberty or as they age, even though frequently at a slower and less sizable fee than ladies.

Chapter 1

The correlation between women, hormones, and meals.

Hormones and Food Go Hand in Hand How we assume, feel, and look are all ruled more often than not using our hormones. Especially after the age of 35, hormone imbalance becomes trouble for ladies, who do not produce the same hormones or have the identical speedy metabolism as once they had been in their 20s. However, simply the fact girls have crossed that age threshold or have hormonal issues like endocrine disorder does not mean they are a misplaced motive. The key to balancing your hormones is to be aware of what you eat. Every unmarried factor you consume impacts the balance of your hormones, the features of your blood vessels, the energy of your immune system, and the health of your intestine and apprehensive machine.

Talking approximately about women hormones, Estrogen and progesterone are the most important intercourse hormones in the human body. Estrogen is the hormone responsible for intercourse characteristics and reproductive capabilities in women. Progesterone is the hormone that plays an assisting position within the menstrual cycle and being pregnant.

When you have low tiers of estrogen and progesterone, together with at some point of menopause, it can negatively affect your temper, sexual choice, bone health, and greater.

In this ebook, we can explore ways to enhance estrogen to your frame, as well as whilst it's time to see a physician for low estrogen. Many of those remedies either immediately aid the advent of estrogen or mirror the activity of estrogen within the body.

Food

1. Soybeans

Soybeans and the products made out of them, consisting of tofu and miso, are a top-notch supply of phytoestrogensTrusted Source. Phytoestrogens mimic estrogen in the frame by binding to estrogen receptors and may have estrogenic or anti-estrogenic results. It became revealed that soy can lessen the chance of having breast cancers, it changed into a position that better soy consumption turned linked to a decreased hazard of breast cancer demise. This can be due to the estrogen-like advantages of phytoestrogens.

More huge research is needed on soy and its effects on estrogen degrees inside the body.

2. Flax seeds

Flax seeds also comprise high quantities of phytoestrogens. The primary phytoestrogens in flax are referred to as lignans, which are useful in estrogen metabolism; it's regarded that a flaxseed-rich diet became capable of reducing ovarian most cancers severity and frequency in hens. More human studies are still wished.

3. Sesame seeds

Sesame seeds are another nutritional source of phytoestrogens, research indicates the impact of soybean and sesame oils on rats with estrogen deficiency.

The researchers discovered that a 2-month food regimen supplemented with those oils was able to enhance bone fitness markers. This research suggests a wonderful estrogen-like effect of each sesame and soy seed, even though further human studies are wanted.

Vitamins and minerals

4. Vitamin B

B vitamins play a crucial position in the advent and activation of estrogen within the frame. Low degrees of these vitamins can cause reduced levels of estrogen. Compared ranges of certain B nutrients to breast most cancers danger in premenopausal ladies. Results indicated that better ranges of nutrients B-2 and B-6 have been related to a lower hazard of breast cancer, which can be due to the effect of these vitamins on estrogen metabolism.

5. Vitamin D

Vitamin D features as a hormone inside the frame. It turned out that both nutrition D and estrogen paintings together to lessen the risk of cardiovascular disorder.

The link among these hormones is because of the position that vitamin D plays in estrogen synthesis. This suggests a potential advantage of nutrition D supplementation in low estrogen levels.

6. Boron

Boron is a trace mineral that has a diffusion of roles in the frame. It's been researched for its advantages in lowering the chance of certain sorts of cancer. Boron is likewise necessary for the metabolism of the intercourse hormones testosterone and estrogen.

Researchers accept as true that boron influences estrogen receptors by allowing the body to extra without problems using the estrogen available.

7. DHEA.

DHEA, or dehydroepiandrosterone, is a certainly occurring hormone that can be transformed into estrogen and testosterone. Within the frame, DHEATrusted Source is first transformed to androgens after which further transformed to estrogens.

One study trusted Source additionally discovered that DHEA can be capable of providing similar advantages within the frame as estrogen.

Herbal dietary supplements

8. Black cohosh

Black cohosh is a traditional Native American herb that has traditionally been used to deal with a selection of conditions, such as menopause and menstrual issues.

Researchers trust that black cohosh additionally consists of positive compounds that stimulate estrogen receptors. Although extra research remains needed, this can propose a possible gain of black cohosh dietary supplements while estrogen is low.

9. Chasteberry

Chasteberry is a conventional herbal treatment that's most widely known for its use in gynecological conditions, which include PMS. Researchers reviewed the to-be-had literature for the Vitex species, which includes chaste berry. They discovered that it became capable of showing off estrogenic outcomes on the dosages of 0.6 and 1.2 grams/kilogram of body weight.

These advantages most probably come from a phytoestrogen in chaste berry known as apigenin.

10. Evening primrose oil

Evening primrose oil (EPO) is a traditional natural remedy that contains excessive tiers of omega-6 fatty acids, making it a popular complement for situations inclusive of PMS and menopause. There are very few current studies on the advantages of evening primrose oil for estrogen.

However, Researchers determined that of over 2,2 hundred ladies that used EPO after discontinuing hormone replacement therapy, 889 stated EPO as useful for controlling the symptoms of low estrogen with menopause.

11. Red clover.

Red clover is a natural supplement that contains a handful of plant compounds known as isoflavones that can act like estrogen inside the body. These isoflavones encompass:

biochanin A

formononetin

genistein

daidzein

Researchers examined the effect of pink clover on hot flashes and hormone levels in women. The researchers located 4 research that confirmed a large increase in estrogen ranges with red clover dietary supplements.

12. Dong Quai.

Dong Quai is a traditional Chinese medicinal drug typically taken for the symptoms of menopause. Like the alternative herbal dietary supplements above, dong Quai carries compounds that function as phytoestrogens.

Researchers examined the feasible estrogenic compounds in 17 famous herbal dietary supplements. They observed viable compounds in Dong Quai that exhibit estrogenic activity.

Ways to enhance progesterone naturally

In many cases, when you have low estrogen you would possibly also have low progesterone. This is specially not unusual during menopause when most of the lady's hormones drop appreciably.

Progesterone is normally boosted thru lotions and medicines, however, a few may additionally decide upon an extra herbal approach.

One feasible manner to boost progesterone is through natural supplements. One study trusted Source observed that chaste berry became capable of improving mid-cycle progesterone levels. However, not all herbal supplements are powerful for reinforcing progesterone. Another study trusted by sources discovered that a couple of Chinese natural medication supplements in reality diminished progesterone degrees.

A better way to naturally enhance progesterone tiers is through a healthy diet and lifestyle. Eating numerous weight-reduction plans can offer the frame the nutrients it needs for progesterone metabolism.

This includes ingredients consisting of cruciferous veggies, nuts, and whole grains. Keeping a healthy weight, staying on a regular sleep timetable, and dealing with strain can help to hold hormones balanced as properly. If natural isn't enough

Natural interventions might not be powerful for every person. Certain humans are extremely touchy about the signs of low estrogen, which include:

hot flashes

mood swings

painful sex

depression

When those signs and symptoms intervene with each day's existence and herbal methods aren't assisting, there are scientific remedies to be had.

Hormone replacement remedy: is a not unusual treatment for menopause. It entails replacing estrogen and progesterone through:
pictures
drugs
lotions
vaginal suppositories

The risks of hormone replacement remedy encompass an expanded hazard of:
blood clots
cardiovascular ailment
stroke
breast cancer
Too a good deal of estrogen, also known as estrogen dominance, may be caused by an expansion of factors. Some ladies naturally produce extra estrogen than progesterone. Supplementation for low estrogen can also cause this form of hormonal imbalance.

The signs and symptoms of high estrogen in ladies include:
bloating

irregular intervals

temper swings

tension

memory troubles

Men also can experience estrogen dominance, which provides gynecomastia, erectile disorder, and infertility.

Chapter 2

What Should I Eat To Balance My Hormones?

The Anatomy Of A Hormone Balancing Plate

While we talked in advance about how reducing positive foods can have a bad impact on the endocrine gadget, it's also possible to over consume 'appropriate' foods, which is why it is important to consume a varied, balanced eating regimen. This will ensure that your body gets the nourishment it desires to maintain a healthy endocrine device, assist your hormones to function optimally, and hold practical body weight.

We have prepared the right anatomy of a hormone balancing plate one which includes the encouraged amounts of the crucial foods which you need for sustaining true hormone function.

This plate must incorporate a third to a half of veggies, which include cruciferous veggies, 30% whole grains, 20% lean protein, and 10% fats. While it can not be viable to get the percentages right for each meal, you ought to intend to consume those food organizations in their respective chances every day.

Organic Fruit And Vegetables

Non-natural produce can comprise pesticides such as glyphosate, which act as hormone disruptors, negatively affecting fertility. Buy natural wherein feasible, and look out for non-GMO ingredients, as these are exposed to less glyphosate.

It may be costly to shop for the most effective natural meals, which is why the 'grimy dozen' listing became created – that is a list of fruit and greens that must most effective be fed on organically, as they're more at risk of absorbing pesticides, but it additionally info produce that it isn't essential to consume natural if sources do not permit.

Alongside consuming nature, it's also crucial to avoid shopping for meals that are plastic-wrapped. Bisphenols in difficult plastics (which include ingesting straws and water bottles) and phthalates in gentle and flexible plastics are endocrine disruptors, and because of this they interfere with the everyday functioning of the endocrine system. Use glass, paper, or different herbal substances to save your ingredients, if feasible, and honestly keep away from microwaveable food, because the plastic consists of toxic chemical compounds which leach into the food all through the microwaving procedure.

Prebiotic And Probiotic Foods

The intestine now not only produces positive hormones but also detoxifies hormones together with estrogen. Therefore, it is vital to nourish your intestine with prebiotic and probiotic ingredients, which can be designed to adjust the intestine microbiome (the gathering of microorganisms that live in the gut).

Probiotics are live pathogens that can be consumed to benefit the intestines. They are often discovered in fermented ingredients, consisting of yogurt, miso, kefir, sauerkraut, kombucha, and kimchi. Prebiotics are fed on with the aid of probiotics to inspire growth and hobby. These consist of garlic, asparagus, banana, leek, tomato, and oats. Probiotics are the best microorganisms that reside inside the gut, while prebiotics are fibrous foods that allow microorganisms to flourish. The gut is the biggest endocrine organ inside the body and synthesizes and secretes greater than 20 hormones that play a position in appetite, satiety, and metabolism. Smith recommends consuming prebiotic ingredients like uncooked garlic and oats, asparagus, dandelion, almonds, apples, bananas, Jerusalem artichokes, and chicory. Absorb probiotics like kimchi and yogurt too.

Phytoestrogens

Phytoestrogens are dietary estrogens that are found in certain flowers. They can modulate estrogen, so whether you're in an estrogen dominant or deficient nation, they'll be beneficial in your weight loss program. Sources of phytoestrogens include flaxseed, chia seed, fennel, lentils, pulses, alfalfa sprouts, and licorice. Soy additionally incorporates a phytoestrogen known as isoflavone, which could decrease your chance of ischemic heart disorder as well as relieve hot flashes.

Good Fats

Omega-3 fatty acids cannot be produced by the body, so it's crucial to include them in a balanced eating regimen. Foods that incorporate omega-three encompass flaxseed, chia seeds, more virgin olive oil, and avocados. Fatty fish is also an extraordinary source, with the most effective being those in the 'SMASH' acronym: sardines, mackerel, anchovies, salmon, and herring.

Omega-6 is also vital for cellular features. However, it could be overconsumed in a food regimen that is high in fried or processed foods. It is important to maintain a balance between omega-3 and omega-6; consequently processed ingredients should get replaced with healthier alternatives such as nuts, chicken, eggs, and seeds.

Cruciferous Vegetables

As nice as being complete with antioxidants that guard your frame against free radicals, cruciferous greens additionally have beneficial consequences on estrogen metabolism, mainly fighting estrogen dominance.

Cruciferous greens are any vegetable inside the Brassica own family, which incorporates cauliflower, broccoli, kale, and brussels sprouts.

However, the highest tiers of sulforaphane (the compound observed in cruciferous veggies that encourages estrogen detoxing) can be found in broccoli sprouts, which can be easy to develop at home on the windowsill.

A Recipe For Hormone Balancing

Stuck for ideas on what to consume to improve your hormone stability? Here is a delicious recipe for a clean, zingy salmon and cauliflower salad, with evidently detoxifying black rice.

Salmon And Cauliflower Salad
Ingredients:
80g black rice, rinsed
1 pink onion
1 cauliflower
1 tbsp more virgin olive oil
2 small salmon fillets
1 avocado
Juice one lime, plus extra wedges to serve
1 small garlic clove, crushed

2 tsp honey

25g mint leaves, shredded

Method

- Wash the rice and cook consistently with the pack instructions. Preheat the oven to 200°C (gasoline mark 6).
- Slice the onion into wedges and reduce the cauliflower into small florets.
- Line a baking tray with parchment paper, and vicinity the onion and cauliflower on top. Drizzle with 1/2 the olive oil, then season with salt and pepper. Toss to mix. Cook for 15 minutes, and change it over.
- Prepare the salmon fillets with seasoning, then add them to the tray of vegetables in the oven and cook collectively for some other 15 minutes, or till the fish is cooked.
- Cut the avocado in half, then scrape the flesh right into a bowl and discard the seed and pores and skin.
- Mash the flesh with the fork again or fork to the desired consistency, then upload a teaspoon of lime juice and mix.

- In a larger bowl, blend the relaxation of the olive oil with the ultimate lime juice, garlic, and honey.
- Stir the rice into this bowl whilst it has cooked, draining any leftover water ahead. When the rice is done, dry then add to the bowl and stir.
- Take the tray out of the oven, then add the cauliflower, crimson onion, and shredded mint to the bowl and toss to mix.
- Divide between two plates. Flake the salmon fillets with a fork, then place them on a pinnacle of the salad.
- Serve each component with a scoop of smashed avocado and a wedge of lime to squeeze on top.

Begin Your Hormone Balancing Journey

When considering hormone balancing, your weight loss plan is simply one part of a holistic approach.

When we reflect on what to eat to nourish our bodies, hormones won't usually be at the top of our thoughts. But our hormones play a completely essential position in our bodies. Hormones are chemical messengers which might be part of the endocrine machine and assist with growth and improvement, metabolism and digestion, fertility, pressure and temper, and extra.

When hormones get out of balance too much or too little are produced or something interferes with signaling pathways it can result in troubles like diabetes, weight loss or advantage, or infertility, amongst other issues.

A healthy food regimen can help maintain hormones in form. Here's an overview of what your hormones manage and which foods keep them balanced.

How a weight loss plan impacts hormones
What we eat influences the production of hormones and their signaling pathways. "Our hormones like healthy fats, like olive oil, avocado, nuts, and seeds, as well as sufficient fiber from fruits and vegetables and high-quality proteins like eggs, fish and meat, hormone, and fertility dietitian at Avocado Grove Nutrition. In contrast, pesticides, alcohol, and artificial sweeteners can negatively impact hormones. You need enough calories too. Female bodies especially are very sensitive to shortage. If your body would not sense that it is getting sufficient, it downregulates the manufacturing of sex hormones. Your frame doesn't understand the difference between a battle or famine or a new weight-loss weight-reduction plan you are following.

How to understand if hormones are imbalanced

During reproductive years, ladies can look to their cycle to provide the signs and symptoms that their hormones are out of the stable. Infertility, 'length problems' like PMS, heavy, painful intervals, and migraines all can be signs and symptoms that hormones are out of stability. Sudden weight fluctuations or changes in power stages can also signal a hormonal imbalance. But, truly, the great way to recognize positives is to get tested.

How hormones works In our body

There are over 2 hundred hormones inside the body. Estrogen, testosterone, cortisol, insulin, leptin, ghrelin, and thyroid hormones are the most commonly known. These are related carefully to metabolism, fertility, and mood.

Metabolism

Insulin: Insulin is released from the pancreas once you consume and takes sugar (glucose) from the blood to cells for energy. Insulin is likewise the hormone accountable for storing extra sugar as fat.

Leptin: This is launched from fat cells and helps manipulate the urge for food, hold weight and inform the brain you're complete. It's often called the "satiety hormone."

Ghrelin: This hormone is liable for stimulating your appetite and is often referred to as the "hunger hormone."

Thyroid hormones: Triiodothyronine (T3) and thyroxine (T4) help adjust weight, power, temperature, the boom of hair, skin, and nails, and more.

Reproductive System

Estrogen: This is the girl intercourse hormone that ends in modifications for the duration of puberty and enables to alter the menstrual cycle, keep the pregnancy, preserve cholesterol in tests and hold bones strong.

Testosterone: The male sex hormone that results in modifications throughout puberty; increases sex force, bone density, and muscle electricity (in both ladies and men).

Stress and Mood

Cortisol: Cortisol is released in instances of pressure and increases blood pressure and heart price. Too much is not right for your health, and it is regularly referred to as the "pressure hormone."

Adrenaline: Our "combat or flight" hormone is launched in instances of strain and will increase coronary heart fee.

Melatonin: This hormone is released at night and prepares the frame for sleep. It's regularly referred to as our "sleep-inducing hormone."

Best ingredients for hormone balance

Cruciferous vegetables

"Cruciferous veggies, in particular broccoli and broccoli sprouts, are superstars at helping our livers metabolize estrogen in a green and healthful way," says Brammer. Cauliflower, Brussels sprouts, kale, and cabbage with bok choy are cruciferous veggies too. "Consuming them frequently is one way to shield yourself from developing estrogen-dominant cancers," says Brammer. Roast them with a drizzle of olive oil, which helps growth absorption of nutrients A, D, E K, or attempt them in our broccoli-cauliflower soup.

Salmon and albacore tuna

Saturated fats are the building blocks of hormones. You need sufficient cholesterol to make intercourse hormones like estrogen and testosterone. The key is to select fat excessive in omega-3s and to limit saturated fats (and remove trans fat). Salmon, canned albacore tuna, walnuts, flaxseed, olive oil, avocados, and chia seeds are excessive in omega-3 fatty acids.

Salmon additionally stabilizes your hunger hormones and is high in diet D, which facilitates regulate female testosterone ranges," says Carrie Gabriel M.S., RDN, a dietitian and owner of Steps Nutrition. "The desirable fat in fish enhances universal hormonal conversation. The endocrine device makes use of hormones to speak with the brain, which in turn boosts our temper and offers us higher cognitive competencies."

Avocados

"Avocados are loaded with beta-sitosterol, which may undoubtedly affect blood cholesterol levels and assist stability cortisol. The plant sterols in avocados also have an impact on estrogen and progesterone, the 2 hormones accountable for regulating ovulation and menstrual cycles." A look at where the combination of fat and fiber in avocados improved hormones that sell satiety, which includes peptide YY (PYY), cholecystokinin (CCK), and glucagon-like peptide 1 (GLP-1). Add half an avocado to breakfast or lunch that will help you live completely for hours, or use avocado in those healthful avocado recipes.

Fruits and greens (preferably natural)

"There is research that shows that even one serving of a high-pesticide fruit or vegetable (consisting of strawberries) has a bad impact on fertility, Many insecticides act as hormone disruptors, meaning they either mimic hormones in your body or they affect the moves of your hormones. The benefits of ingesting results and veggies some distance outweigh not consuming them if you cannot manage to pay to devour organic. Minimize publicity if you can, however , realize that each fruit and greens are wealthy in vitamins, minerals, and antioxidants. Consider shopping natural from the "Dirty Dozen" list, which is a ranking of the most infected produce from the Environmental Working Group.

High-fiber carbohydrates

Think culmination, greens, and complete grains. "Eating an eating regimen excessive in fiber can assist clean excess hormones from the frame. Fiber, as well as lignans, which can be ample in flaxseed, facilitate binding and elimination of unbound energetic estrogens. Focus on making 1/2 of your plate non starchy vegetables at most food and a fourth of your plate starchy vegetables like potatoes or whole grains. "Root veggies like carrots, candy potatoes, and squashes can be beneficial, together with entire grains and beans. Including a few starches at dinner can also assist to adjust the hormones melatonin and cortisol too. a few carbs can help to mitigate improved cortisol degrees.

Worst foods for hormone stability

Eat less processed ingredients, fried ingredients, sugar, and artificial sweeteners, and drink less alcohol to avoid hormone imbalances.

Research indicates that downing artificial sweeteners may additionally regulate our intestine bacteria, which might also impact the stability of starvation and satiety, the one's equal hormones leptin and ghrelin.

Alcohol interferes with several hormonal strategies, from blood sugar control to estrogen metabolism. Booze is associated with a multiplied hazard for breast cancers, in addition to other cancers. Stick to no multiple drinks a day in case you're a lady and no more than beverages in step with the day if you're a person.

Stress, sleep, and exercise

In addition to a healthy food regimen, getting ok sleep, keeping pressure levels low and workout frequently is all essential for hormone balance.

Sleep deprivation is linked to low testosterone in men, and lack of sleep interferes with leptin and ghrelin (consequently, why you tend to crave carbs and all the snacks when you're tired). Chronic stress leads to expanded levels of cortisol, which suppresses the digestive and immune systems and might motivate excessive blood stress. Cortisol also results in carb cravings. Exercise, meditation, sleep, and ingesting chocolate enhance degrees of norepinephrine and serotonin. Norepinephrine boosts power, and serotonin is the "sense exact" hormone.

Chapter 3

HOW DOES FOOD AFFECT YOUR HORMONES?

We have all heard the phrase 'meals is gas' – however what does that mean? A bit like a vehicle, we want gas for you. However, whilst motors require petrol or diesel, we require meals! So, how does food affect our hormones? Food offers the vitamins we need to hold wholesome frame structures, including the manufacturing, metabolism, and detoxing of hormones. Therefore, if we don't get enough of the proper nutritious foods, our hormone stability can suffer.

Why Does Food Have Effects On Hormones?

There are around 2 hundred distinctive hormones inside the human body. These are chemical messengers that manipulate several structures, which include our metabolism, the immune system, menstrual cycle, and duplicate. Consuming sure ingredients can provide the nutrients that we need to facilitate the production of hormones.

How Does Food Affect Hormones? An Important Example

Steroid hormones – inclusive of testosterone, estrogen, and progesterone – contribute to the normal characteristic of all the above structures and extra. They are many of the most important and energetic hormones within the body. But did you understand that they're synthesized from LDL cholesterol?

Dr. Ghazala Aziz-Scott, Hormone Specialist at the Marion Gluck Clinic explains: "Unfortunately, LDL cholesterol has an awful reputation due to the fact having high stages in your blood can cause cholesterol plaque building up, furring the arteries and leading to coronary heart sickness. However, having too little cholesterol also can negatively affect your body. For example, ladies who've extremely low body fats can also suffer from a scarcity of periods (amenorrhea) and infertility. This is because there isn't enough LDL cholesterol for the frame to synthesize estrogen and progesterone, which might be essential hormones within the reproductive machine.

Utmost Dieting And The Effects On The Hormones.

Due to food containing cholesterol, as well as different undeservedly notorious meal corporations consisting of carbohydrates being portrayed so poorly within the media, we've seen the emergence of diets that reduce those foods completely, which includes low fat and keto. Often, these diets are unsustainable, cutting out major food agencies over some time for an 'instant weight loss solution'. Most of the time, individuals who adopt those diets locate that they put weight back following the cease of the diet, as the frame clings onto its power assets in case of some other period of nutrient hunger- the so-called yo-yo dieting syndrome.

Not handiest that, but the effect of an excessive weight-reduction plan may have an extensive impact on the endocrine gadget. Instead of following an intense or crash diet, the focus needs to be on preserving a sustainable weight-reduction plan filled with nutritious, unprocessed whole foods from a huge range of meal groups. Below, we've indexed the nutrients and meals that should be protected in a nicely-rounded food plan that can maintain balanced hormone stages.

Chapter 4

How to assist hormones and universal health as you age

So, what do you need to do with all of these facts? While hormone stages certainly change over time, there are some steps you can take to lessen the effect.

1. Work along with your health practitioner to find alleviation from tough signs

Learning to be aware of your frame early on so that you can be aware of any changes can be key to figuring out problems before they get out of manipulation. The outcomes of hormonal adjustments differ from individual to man or woman. For some, it may be a minor concern, while for others it can be of such importance that it causes disruptions to the daily dwelling. Symptoms together with weight fluctuations, fatigue, persistent joint ache, low libido, heart fee fluctuations, modifications in bowel actions, or even despair are some that must be regarded as a way to contact your scientific company.

2. Adopt a Mediterranean-fashion eating regimen

With the herbal growth in infection that occurs as you age, it is useful and scrumptious to contain the ideas of the Mediterranean weight loss program. This way of ingesting has been praised for its capability to assist shield your coronary heart and mind as you age, decrease the chance for diabetes, and make losing weight and keeping a healthy weight less difficult and much greater. And in contrast to maximum diets, it would not advocate aside from anybody specific meals or food groups.

When people think about ingredients affecting their body, they generally tend to be aware of what they need to stop ingesting instead of the things they may no longer be ingesting sufficient. For example, carbohydrates are often frowned upon, particularly as part of present-day weight loss diets, but what people don't know is that carbohydrates are "essential for a healthful reproductive hormone reaction," similarly to just about every other bodily function. And your body desires LDL cholesterol and fats to accurately produce hormones, so it's critical to pay attention to incorporating healthful sources of fat into your weight-reduction plan as properly.

And first-class of all, the Mediterranean eating regimen is simple to follow, which enables reduce down on lifestyle pressure.

3. Watch out for hormone-disrupting chemical substances

The pollutants you're uncovered inside the environment also play a main role in hormone fitness. Chemicals referred to as xenoestrogens can mimic or even trade the actions of our hormones. To a defensive degree, she recommends proscribing publicity to hormone-disrupting chemical substances, such as plastics made with BPA (bisphenol A) and phthalates, and pesticides, in addition to pure beauty and cleaning merchandise that comprises ingredients like triclosan.

4. Decrease stress

We all know how destructive strain may be on our fitness. And because cortisol levels grow as we age, we're going to need to fight that stress thru a healthful eating regimen and lifestyle conduct, even as also operating to cast off assets of strain from our lives wherein we can.

5. Incorporate energy education

Despite what you may think, aerobics isn't everything. While it's vital to get your coronary heart pumping with cozy-to-you aerobic sporting activities, because muscle tissues and bone density decrease as we age, incorporating energy education can be even greater useful.

The bottom line here is that some hormone modifications are a natural part of growing older, and at the same time as some symptoms may be uncomfortable to deal with, there are methods to assist mitigate their impact. And remember, it's constantly an awesome concept to speak with your medical doctor about any concerning symptoms.

Chapter 5

Different herbs can stabilize a woman's hormones?

There are many herbs to stabilize girl hormones. Herbs are a remarkable manner to balance female hormones certainly. Here are 8 herbs to stability lady hormones:

1. Vitex to balance lady hormones

Vitex, additionally known as chaste berry, is used to deal with a diffusion of various conditions, including PMS, infertility, pimples, and more. It is a perfect herb to stabilize girl hormones. Vitex works by reducing tiers of prolactin, which in turn balances out estrogen and progesterone. Chasteberry can be observed in teas or supplements.

2. Raspberry Leaf to balance girl hormones

Raspberry leaf tea is a not unusual herb to stabilize girl hormones. The plant compound in pink raspberry leaves may additionally have antioxidant effects and may help to relax blood vessels. These compounds might also have a muscle relaxation effect, depending on the quantity consumed, making them useful for menstrual cramps in a few girls. Red raspberry leaf tea is likewise regularly used throughout late pregnancy to support labor and delivery.

3. Black cohosh to stability woman hormones

Black cohosh is frequently used to treat menopause signs and symptoms consisting of hot flashes, moodiness, excessive sweating, and more. It also has use in inducing hard work in pregnant ladies, premenstrual syndrome (PMS), and dysmenorrhea (or painful periods). Black cohosh is an extraordinary herb to balance women's hormones due to the fact it's far a phytoestrogen, that can assist to decrease accelerated estrogen or boost low estrogen. Black cohosh is regularly discovered in a complementing shape. It isn't really useful to use at some point of being pregnant or breastfeeding

4. Dong Quai to stability woman's hormones

Dong Quai, also referred to as woman ginseng, is an herb commonly utilized in traditional Chinese remedies. It has been used for hundreds of years as an herb to balance female hormones and save you symptoms of PMS. Dong Quai has been shown to balance degrees of estrogen, which in go back alleviates common symptoms of menopause or PMS. It can be found in complementary shapes or you could even buy dong quai tea.

5. *Fenugreek seed to balance female hormones*
Fenugreek seed incorporates phytoestrogens, which assist balance estrogen, making it a notable herb to balance lady hormones. Studies show that fenugreek may assist painful periods (or dysmenorrhea). This herb may additionally assist to increase low testosterone and improve low libido in girls. Fenugreek can be observed in tea, supplements, or spices.

6. *Dandelion root to stability female hormones*
Dandelion root is excessive in plant estrogens and plays a sizable position in the cleansing of

the frame, which plays a crucial role in detoxifying excess hormones in the frame. This herb might also help to save you from constipation, which is a critical step in clearing hormones from the frame. It can be determined in tea or dietary supplements.

7. Cramp bark to balance girl hormones

Cramp bark is an herb that helps reduce menstrual cramps. It acts as a muscle relaxer, decreasing the pain of menstrual cramps. Those struggling with PMS signs or painful cramps ought to enjoy the muscle relaxant outcomes of cramp bark.

8. Ginger Rhizome to balance female hormones

Ginger rhizome is any other call for ginger and it's far an extraordinary herb to balance girl hormones. Ginger has been used as a spice and for its many medicinal residences. Ginger has a ton of anti-inflammatory homes and is generally used to treat nausea. Ginger reduces the production of prostaglandins, which in turn reduces commonplace signs and symptoms associated with PMS including cramps, temper swings, and complications. Ginger may be found in teas, dietary supplements, or spices, or you could even upload a chunk of ginger to your smoothies for a nice kick of flavor.

So, how does food affect our hormones? Food gives the nutrients we want to keep healthful body systems, which include the production, metabolism, and detoxification of hormones. Therefore, if we don't get enough of the right nutritious meals, our hormone stability can suffer.